# Paleo for Beginners

## *The 7-Day Paleo Diet Plan for Maximum Nutrition, Weight Loss and Achieving Vibrant Health*

By

Anne Wilson

# Table of Contents

# Introduction

I want to thank you and congratulate you for purchasing the book, *"Paleo for Beginners: The 7-Day Paleo Diet Plan for Maximum Nutrition, Weight Loss and Achieving Vibrant Health"*.

This book contains proven steps and strategies on how to create mouthwatering dishes that will surely help you start on your paleo diet marvelously.

People who wanted to explore the paleo diet as well as those who are just starting in it will surely find this book a great help. It has a list of all food products that are considered paleo as well as those that are not.

Knowing what you can eat and what you can't will give you a general idea on the kind of meals you'll usually have. It can also remove some of the apprehensions that you may be feeling developing new eating habits. Once you get more familiar with what's accepted and what's not, you may be able to re-create recipes of your favorite dishes to make them paleo-friendly. You may even find yourself creating new ones!

In this book, you will find a 7-day meal plan to help you start on your paleo diet as well as recipes to allow you to create the dishes. These dishes are not only nutritious but are also easy to make and incredibly delicious.

You may run into trouble regarding condiments once you go paleo. Undeniably, condiments add more flavor to your food but the ones that you can buy in stores may contain ingredients that are not accepted in paleo. A final chapter is added into this book containing paleo-approved recipes for condiments. With it, you wouldn't have to worry about your food tasting bland.

Thanks again for purchasing this book, I hope you enjoy it!

# CHAPTER 1

# Paleo or Not Paleo? That is the Question

## What is Considered Paleo?

Meats are generally accepted in the paleo diet. Just make sure to avoid meat products that contain large amounts of fat such as hot dogs and spam as well as highly processed meats. Feel free to eat beef, wild boar, chicken, quail, pork, bison, lamb, horse, veal, sheep, goose and goat.

You can also consume game meats such as deer, wild turkey, pheasant, reindeer, bear, rabbit, moose, duck, woodcock and elk. Eggs from chicken, goose, duck and quail are also included in this diet.

Fishes are good sources of protein and omega 3. You can still enjoy eating salmon, herring, tuna, anchovy, walleye, trout, mackerel, bass, grouper, halibut, flatfish, sole, cod, haddock, tilapia and turbot even if you go on a paleo diet.

Aside from fishes, other types of seafood such as crab, oysters, crawfish, scallops, crayfish, lobster, shrimp and clams are also included in this food regimen.

Your body uses fats as an energy source thus it is important that your body contains enough amounts of it. Avocado oil, tallow, coconut milk, olive oil, nut butters, coconut oil, lamb fat, butter, veal fat, ghee, duck fat, lard and nut oils such as macadamia and walnut are some of the accepted fats in the paleo diet.

Paleo dishes are extremely healthy as they usually contain good amounts of vegetables. Once you start going paleo, expect to see more of plant products such as celery, okra, peppers, artichokes, onions, broccoli, Brussels sprouts, leeks, cabbage, kohlrabi, cucumber, eggplants, asparagus, squash and cauliflower.

Green leafy vegetables such as lettuce, radicchio, spinach, chicory, collard greens, rapini, kale, arugula and watercress are also accepted. In addition, carrots, cassava, beets, yams, turnips, radishes, parsnips, sweet potatoes, rutabaga and other root vegetables are included in paleo diet.

Fruits are also considered as paleo food but they may contain huge amounts of fructose. It would be best to limit your daily fruit consumption to a maximum of 3 servings especially if you are aiming to lose weight. Bananas, apples, oranges, berries, pears, coconut, peaches, tangerine, nectarines, mango, plums, lime, pineapple, lemon, grapes, melon, cantaloupe, watermelon, apricot and cherries are some of the most commonly used fruits in paleo recipes.

Pistachios, hazelnuts, Brazil nuts, almonds, pecans, cashews, walnuts, chestnuts, pine nuts, macadamia nuts and other kinds of nuts are also included in the list of accepted food in paleo. Mushrooms, herbs, edible plant seeds and spices are also considered paleo-friendly.

**Warning: Not Paleo**

Once you start on your paleo diet, you should say goodbye to dairy products. These include, but are not limited to, cheese, ice cream, cottage cheese, milk, dairy creamer, yogurt, dairy spreads and cream cheese.

Products that contain high amounts of sugar such as soft drinks and candies are also banned from this diet. Anything that is made artificially such as artificial sweeteners and energy drinks are also not included in the paleo diet. Honey and maple syrup can be used to sweeten your food instead.

Grains are also not included in the paleo menu. The same is true for any food product that may contain grains such as cereals, pasta, bread, beer, hash browns, corn syrup and pancakes. If you love eating these kinds of food before, you don't have to worry about going paleo. There are paleo-approved recipes for these so you can still enjoy them without straying away from your diet.

Beans, peas, peanuts, lentils, soybeans and other types of legumes are also not considered paleo-friendly. The same goes for any food containing them.

# CHAPTER 2

# Day One

## *Breakfast: Spinach Quiche*

Number of Servings: 3

### *Ingredients:*

5 large eggs

½ teaspoon baking powder

1 clove garlic, minced

1 ½ cups fresh spinach, chopped

½ cup coconut milk

½ medium onion, chopped

Ground black pepper

Sea salt

### *Instructions:*

a. Set the oven to 350 degrees.

b. Combine coconut milk and eggs together in a large bowl. Mix well.

c. Add remaining ingredients while whisking coconut milk mixture continuously.

d. Use a non-stick cooking spray to grease a 9-inch pie dish.

e. Pour the coconut milk mixture into the pie dish and place it in the oven.

f. Cook for about 30 minutes.

# Lunch: Sun-dried Tomato Roulade

Number of Servings: 4

## Ingredients:

4 cutlets turkey

4 tablespoon olive oil

7 sun-dried tomatoes

2 tablespoons pine nuts

½ teaspoon sea salt

20 leaves basil

Black pepper

Sea salt

Coconut oil

## Instructions:

a. Set the oven to 350 degrees.

b. Put pine nuts in a skillet and place it over medium-high heat. Toast for about 4 minutes. Shake occasionally.

c. Once done, transfer nuts into a food processor. Add basil, tomatoes and salt. Blend well.

d. Add olive oil into the mixture while being processed.

e. Place each cutlet in a plate and sprinkle with salt. Distribute the tomato mixture into each cutlet evenly.

f.  Roll each cutlet tightly. Secure in place using a toothpick.

g.  Using a medium skillet, cook the roulade in coconut oil over medium-high heat until brown on both sides.

h.  Transfer the pan into the oven and bake for 10 minutes.

# *Dinner: Spaghetti Squash with Mushroom Sauce*

Number of Servings: 4

## *Ingredients:*

1 spaghetti squash

5 cloves garlic, minced

4 oz. pancetta, chopped

1 onion, chopped

1 ¼ cups shiitake mushrooms, chopped

1 cup coconut milk

1 teaspoon dried oregano

2 tablespoons ghee

1 teaspoon onion powder

Ground black pepper

Sea salt

## *Instructions:*

a.  Set the oven to 350 degrees beforehand.

b.  Slice the squash in half lengthwise and scoop out the seeds.

c.  Put the squash slices in a baking pan and place it in the oven. Let it cook for about 30 minutes.

d.  Pour coconut milk into a saucepan together with ghee, oregano, 2 minced garlic cloves and onion powder.

e. Cook sauce over medium-low heat until thick. Stir frequently and season to taste. Once done, set aside.

f. Using a skillet, sauté garlic and onion in extra ghee over medium heat for about 2 minutes.

g. Add mushrooms and pancetta. Once mushrooms are soft, pour sauce into the skillet and stir well. Adjust seasoning as needed.

h. Shred the squash using a fork and pour mushroom sauce on top.

## *Dessert: Pumpkin Pie Pudding*

Number of Servings: 4

### *Ingredients:*

½ cup pumpkin puree, unsweetened

1/8 teaspoon allspice, ground

1 ¾ cups almond milk

¼ teaspoon ginger, ground

¼ cup honey, raw

1 teaspoon vanilla extract

¼ teaspoon nutmeg, ground

2 tablespoons tapioca starch

½ teaspoon cinnamon, ground

1 large egg

1 tablespoon water

### *Instructions:*

a. Dissolve the tapioca starch in water in a small bowl.

b. Put almond milk into a saucepan together with honey and egg. Mix well.

c. Bring mixture into a boil while stirring frequently. Add tapioca mixture while whisking continuously.

d.  Allow to cook for about 2 minutes then remove from heat.

e.  Put all of the remaining ingredients in a bowl and stir well.

f.  Gradually combine the two mixtures together. Place the saucepan back over low heat.

g.  Cook for about 4 minutes. Stir constantly.

h.  Distribute the pudding evenly in dessert bowls. Refrigerate for at least 2 hours.

Additional Tip: For a nut-free version of this recipe, you can use coconut milk instead of almond milk.

# *Snack: Granola Bars*

## *Ingredients:*

4 cups nuts, assorted

1 tablespoon sea salt

1 cup shredded coconut

1 teaspoon cinnamon

1 cup dried fruit

1 teaspoon vanilla extract

1/3 cup coconut oil

¼ cup honey, raw

1/3 cup almond butter

## *Instructions:*

a.  Combine water and salt together in a pot. Put nuts in it and let them soak overnight. Afterwards, drain excess water and rinse well.

b.  Set an oven to 150 degrees beforehand.

c.  Transfer nuts to a baking sheet and arrange them in a single layer.

d.  Place the baking sheet in the oven and allow nuts to roast for 12 hours. Set aside to cool once done.

e.  Divide the nuts into two equal halves. Chop half of the nuts roughly using a knife. Grind remaining nuts into fine grains using a food processor.

f.  Put coconut oil, cinnamon, almond butter, vanilla and honey in a saucepan and place it over medium heat.

g.  Once bubbles form, pour the mixture into a bowl. Add chopped nuts, dried fruit and ground nuts. Mix well.

h.  Transfer the resulting mixture to a baking dish lined with parchment paper. Pack the mixture firmly and tightly.

i.  Allow mixture to set at room temperature for about 2 hours then freeze for an additional hour. Slice into desired size and shape once done.

# CHAPTER 3

# Day Two

## *Breakfast: Red Pepper and Kale Frittata*

Number of Servings: 4

### *Ingredients:*

1 tablespoon coconut oil

½ cup almond milk

½ cup red pepper, chopped

8 large eggs

1/3 cup onion, chopped

2 cups kale

 3 slices crispy bacon, chopped

Ground black pepper

Salt


### *Instructions:*

a.  Set the oven to 350 degrees.

b.  Remove the stems and chop the kale leaves. Season with black pepper and salt. Set aside.

c.  Put almond milk and eggs together in a medium bowl. Stir and combine well.

d.  Using a skillet, sauté red pepper and onions in coconut oil over medium heat for about 3 minutes.

e.  Add kale and let it cook for another 5 minutes.

f.  Pour almond milk mixture into the pan together with bacon. Cook for about 4 minutes.

g.  Place frittata in the oven and bake for about 15 minutes.

Additional Tip: You can use coconut milk as a substitute for almond milk especially if you have food allergies.

# *Lunch: Zucchini Fritters*

Number of Servings: 6

## *Ingredients:*

2 zucchini, shredded

2 tablespoons coconut oil

1 teaspoon sea salt

1 teaspoon black pepper

1 egg

2 tablespoons coconut flour

1 teaspoon cayenne pepper

4 scallions, sliced

## *Instructions:*

a. Combine salt and zucchini together in a bowl. Set aside.

b. Drain excess water from zucchini after 10 minutes and place in another bowl.

c. Add coconut flour, pepper, egg, cayenne and scallions. Mix well.

d. Divide the mixture into 6 equal portions.

e. Using a skillet, cook fritters in coconut oil over medium-high heat until brown on each side.

f. Once done, transfer fritters into a plate lined with paper towels. Sprinkle additional scallions on top.

# *Dinner: Shakshuka*

Number of Servings: 4 to 6

## *Ingredients:*

1 tablespoon ghee

½ tablespoon parsley, chopped finely

½ onion, chopped

6 eggs

2 tablespoons tomato paste

1 clove garlic, minced

1 teaspoon paprika

1 red bell pepper, chopped and seeded

1 teaspoon chili powder

4 cups tomatoes, diced

Cayenne pepper

Ground black pepper

Sea salt

## *Instructions:*

a.  Using a large skillet, sauté onions in ghee over medium heat for about 2 minutes.

b.  Add garlic. Continue cooking until onions are soft and slightly caramelized.

c.  Put bell pepper in the skillet and stir well. Cook for about 5 minutes.

d.  Add tomatoes, cayenne pepper, salt, tomato paste, paprika, black pepper and chili powder and bring mixture to a simmer. Adjust seasoning to your preference and reduce heat as needed.

e.  Break the eggs on top of the mixture with equal spaces in between. Cover and let it cook until eggs are cooked through.

f.  Once done, sprinkle parsley on top.

# *Dessert: Fresh Fruit Popsicle*

Number of Servings: 4

## *Ingredients:*

2 kiwis, sliced and peeled

Coconut water

1 package strawberries, sliced

1 package fresh blueberries

1 package fresh raspberries

## *Instructions:*

a.  Distribute the fresh fruit evenly among popsicle molds.

b.  Pour coconut water into each mold.

c.  Place the molds in the freezer and allow popsicle to set for about 5 hours.

## *Snack: Banana Pumpkin Bread*

### *Ingredients:*

½ cup coconut flour

¾ cup pecans, chopped

½ cup almond flour

½ teaspoon salt

½ cup banana puree

½ teaspoon vanilla extract

½ cup pumpkin puree

4 eggs

½ cup almond butter, melted

¼ cup honey, raw

1 teaspoon baking soda

### *Instructions:*

a. Set an oven to 350 degrees. Grease a loaf pan using a non-stick cooking spray.

b. Place almond flour, baking soda, coconut flour and salt in a bowl. Mix well

c. Put eggs, vanilla extract, butter, pecans, pumpkin puree, honey and banana puree in a separate bowl and stir until smooth.

d. Combine the two mixtures together until well combined.

e.  Transfer the mixture into the loaf pan and place it in an oven.

f.  Bake for about 45 minutes. Set aside for about 10 minutes to cool.

# CHAPTER 4

# Day Three

## *Breakfast: Apple and Cinnamon Waffles*

Number of Servings: 4

### *Ingredients:*

1 ½ cups almond flour

2 tablespoons ghee, melted

¾ teaspoon cinnamon, ground

¼ cup tapioca starch

½ cup coconut milk

1 tablespoon coconut flour

1 tablespoon baking powder

2 eggs

1 granny smith apple, peeled and shredded

1 ½ teaspoon vanilla extract

Sea salt

Fresh fruit slices

## *Instructions:*

a. Heat a waffle iron beforehand.

b. Put almond flour, baking powder, cinnamon, tapioca starch, salt and coconut flour together in a bowl. Mix well.

c. Separate egg yolks from the egg whites.

d. Place egg yolks, ghee, vanilla, apple and coconut milk in a separate bowl and stir well.

e. Combine the two mixtures together in a bowl. Blend until a batter is formed.

f. Using a hand mixer, whisk egg whites until soft peaks are formed.

g. Add egg whites into the batter. Mix gently until thoroughly combined.

h. Grease the waffle iron with extra ghee. Pour the batter into it until completely covered and let it cook for about 3 minutes.

i. Repeat the procedure for the remaining batter.

j. Garnish with fresh fruit slices.

## *Lunch: Butternut Squash and Beef Skillet*

Number of Servings: 3

### *Ingredients:*

2 tablespoons butter

½ avocado, peeled and sliced

450 grams grass fed beef, ground

3 eggs

1 teaspoon cumin, ground

1 small onion, chopped

450 grams spinach, chopped

2 stalks celery, chopped

½ large butternut squash, cooked

3 cloves garlic, minced

1 teaspoon garam masala

½ teaspoon Himalayan salt

½ teaspoon coriander, ground

¼ teaspoon white pepper, ground

## *Instructions:*

a.  Set the oven to 375 degrees

b.  Put the spinach in a microwave and cook for a minute. Once cooled, drain excess moisture and set leaves aside.

c.  Scoop out the flesh of the squash and reserve it for later.

d.  Put butter in a skillet and place it over medium-high heat. Once melted, add onion, garlic and celery into the pan.

e.  Sauté vegetables for about 3 minutes and season with salt.

f.  Add beef, garam masala, white pepper, coriander and cumin.

g.  Continue cooking until beef turns brown then add spinach and squash. Mix well.

h.  Create three hollows in the mixture and crack an egg into each one. Season egg with pepper and salt.

i.  Put the skillet in the oven and let it cook for about 15 minutes.

j.  Once done, remove from the oven. Place avocado on top.

## *Dinner: Chicken Enchilada Casserole*

Number of Servings: 4

### *Ingredients:*

4 cups chicken, cooked and shredded

4 cups mixed greens, chopped

2 bell peppers, diced

1 tomato, diced

1 red onion, diced

1 avocado, diced

6 green onions, sliced thinly

8 oz. tomato sauce

¼ teaspoon onion powder

1 cup water

¼ teaspoon cumin, ground

¼ teaspoon garlic powder

¼ cup chili powder

Ground black pepper

Sea salt

## Instructions:

a. Heat an oven to 375 degrees beforehand.

b. Combine tomato sauce, onion powder, water, garlic powder and cumin together in a sauce pan and place it over medium heat. Season to taste.

c. Allow the sauce to cook for about 10 minutes. Stir occasionally.

d. Place chicken, onions, bell peppers and half of the green onions in a baking dish. Spread enchilada sauce on top and mix thoroughly.

e. Put the baking dish in the oven and let it cook for about 20 minutes. Remove from the oven once done.

f. Distribute mixed greens, avocado, tomato and remaining green onions evenly on top of the mixture.

## *Dessert: Berry Crumble*

Number of Servings: 4

### *Ingredients:*

4 cups mixed fresh berries

½ teaspoon cinnamon, ground

1 cup almond meal

½ cup ghee

1 cup oven-roasted nuts, assorted

### *Instructions:*

a. Set an oven to 350 degrees.

b. Pound the nuts using mortar and pestle or rolling pin into small chunks.

c. Place almond meal, ghee, nuts and cinnamon in a bowl. Mix well.

d. Distribute half of the nut mixture in the bottom of a pie dish. Spread mixed berries on top.

e. Pour remaining nut mixture on top of the berries.

f. Place the pie dish in an oven and cook for about 30 minutes.

# Snack: Raisin Banana Cookies

## Ingredients:

3 bananas, mashed

1 teaspoon cinnamon

¼ cup applesauce

1 teaspoon vanilla

3 cups almond meal

½ cup raisins

½ cup coconut flour

¼ cup full-fat coconut milk

¼ cup coconut flakes

## Instructions:

a. Set the oven to 350 degrees.

b. Combine all of the ingredients together in a bowl. Mix until smooth.

c. Using a spoon, place portions of the mixture in the cookie sheet lined with parchment paper.

d. Bake the cookies for about 30 minutes.

# CHAPTER 5

# Day Four

## *Breakfast: Paleo Burrito*

Number of Servings: 4

### *Ingredients:*

5 eggs, whisked

¼ teaspoon chili flakes

8 slices ham

½ small onion, diced

1 red bell pepper, seeded and diced

1 tomato, seeded and diced

Ground black pepper

Sea salt

Ghee

### *Instructions:*

a.  Using a skillet, sauté onions, chili flakes and bell peppers in ghee over medium-high heat for about 6 minutes.

b.  Add tomatoes into the skillet and cook for another two minutes.

c.  Pour eggs over the vegetables and scramble using a spatula.

d.  Once cooked through, place desired amount of the egg mixture in a slice of ham and roll it up.

e.  Repeat procedure for the remaining ham slices and egg mixture.

f.  Place the ham rolls in the skillet and cook until slightly brown.

## *Lunch: Chicken Pot Pie Skillet*

Number of Servings: 4

### *Ingredients:*

4 cups chicken, cooked and shredded

1 tablespoon fresh dill, minced

4 carrots, sliced

1 cup cremini mushrooms, quartered

2 ¼ cups chicken stock

1 cup red onion, chopped

2 cloves garlic, minced

1 stalk celery, chopped

Ghee

### *Instructions:*

a.  Set the oven to 425 degrees.

b.  Using a skillet, sauté garlic, onion, carrots and celery in ghee over medium-high heat for about 4 minutes.

c.  Add mushrooms into the skillet and cook for additional 4 minutes.

d.  Pour ¼ cup of chicken stock into the mixture. Allow it to cook while scraping the bottom of the pan.

e. Once liquid is reduced by half, add remaining stock together with dill and chicken meat.

f. Cook for about 5 minutes then transfer the skillet into the oven.

g. Bake for about 15 minutes.

# *Dinner: Pesto-Stuffed Tomatoes with Eggs*

Number of Servings: 3 to 4

## *Ingredients:*

6 large tomatoes

3/8 teaspoon ground black pepper

6 eggs

1 clove garlic

½ teaspoon sea salt

½ cup extra virgin olive oil

¼ cup parsley

8 Boston or romaine lettuce leaves

## *Instructions:*

a.  Cut lettuce leaves into small pieces.

b.  Place torn lettuce leaves in a food processor together with garlic, olive oil, parsley, black pepper and salt. Blend until desired consistency is obtained.

c.  Set an oven to 400 degrees beforehand.

d.  Remove the core of the tomatoes including the seeds and pulp. Carefully arrange these in a 9-inch baking dish.

e. Fill each tomato with equal amounts of pesto but keep in mind to allot enough space for the egg.

f. Break an egg into each tomato. Season to taste.

g. Cook the stuffed tomatoes in the oven for about 20 minutes.

# *Dessert: Coconut Squares*

Number of Servings: 4

## *Ingredients:*

3 eggs

¼ teaspoon sea salt

1 cup coconut milk

1 ½ cups unsweetened coconut, shredded

1/3 cup coconut oil

1 tablespoon coconut flour

1/3 cup honey, raw

½ cup almond flour

1 tablespoon vanilla extract

## *Instructions:*

a.  Set the oven to 350 degrees.

b.  Place eggs, vanilla extract, coconut milk, honey and coconut oil together in a bowl. Blend the ingredients using a hand mixer.

c.  Decrease the speed of the hand mixer to the lowest and gradually add almond flour into the mixture.

d.  Add coconut. Continue blending the mixture until a consistent texture is reached.

e.  Distribute the mixture in an 8x8 baking dish evenly and place it in the oven.

f.  Bake for about 30 minutes. Remove from the oven once done and set aside to cool completely. Slice into squares.

# *Snack: Fruit Banana Split*

## *Ingredients:*

2 bananas, sliced lengthwise

1 1/2 cups strawberries, sliced

¼ cup nuts, roasted and chopped

1 ½ cups blueberries

1/3 cup water

¼ cup honey, raw

1 cup raspberries

## *Instructions:*

a. Place water and honey in a saucepan.

b. Add ½ cup of strawberries and ½ cup of blueberries into the pan and mix well.

c. Once mixture starts to boil, reduce the heat and cook gently for about 5 minutes.

d. Using a food processor, blend the sauce until smooth.

e. Place bananas and remaining berries on a plate. Drizzle with the sauce and spread nuts on top.

# CHAPTER 6

# Day Five

## *Breakfast: Paleo Bread*

Number of Servings: 3

### *Ingredients:*

½ tablespoon butter

¼ teaspoon baking soda

1 teaspoon vanilla extract

½ cup roasted almond butter

1 teaspoon cinnamon, ground

2 large eggs

¼ teaspoon k0sher salt

2 tablespoons honey, raw

### *Instructions:*

a.  Set the oven to 325 degrees. Use the butter to grease an 8-inch baking dish.

b.  Put eggs and almond butter in a large bowl. Mix well.

c.  Add vanilla and honey. Stir well.

d. Add cinnamon into the mixture together with baking soda and salt. Blend until ingredients are combined well.

e. Pour the mixture into the baking dish and distribute evenly.

f. Place the baking dish in the oven and let it cook for about 15-20 minutes.

g. Once done, transfer into a cooling rack to cool.

Additional Tip: You can prepare the batter a day before to lessen the time needed to create this dish. Once you have prepared the batter accordingly and transferred it into the baking dish, you'll just have to cover it completely with a plastic wrap before placing it in the refrigerator overnight.

# *Lunch: Asian Beef Stir-Fry*

Number of Servings: 4

## *Ingredients:*

1 ½ lb. steak, sliced thinly

1 hot pepper, sliced

10 oz. snow peas

2 teaspoons apple cider vinegar

10 oz. mushrooms, sliced thinly

½ teaspoon ginger

1/3 cup coconut aminos

6 cloves garlic, minced

2 tablespoons honey

Ghee

Ground black pepper

Sea salt

## *Instructions:*

a. Place coconut aminos, vinegar, honey, ginger and garlic in a bowl. Stir well.

b. Fill a saucepan with water. Once boiling, add peas and cook for about 4 minutes. Once done, remove the peas and reserve for later.

c. Using a skillet, cook mushrooms in ghee over high heat until brown on each side. Remove mushrooms from the pan once done.

d. Place steak in the skillet and cook on each side until brown. Once meat is cooked through, reduce the heat to medium.

e. Add hot pepper and cook for another 2 minutes.

f. Add mushrooms, peas and coconut aminos mixture into the skillet and cook for about 3 minutes. Stir frequently.

# *Dinner: Beef-Stuffed Squash*

Number of Servings: 2

## *Ingredients:*

1 butternut squash, halved and seeded

½ tablespoon cinnamon

1 lb. beef, ground

2 cloves garlic, minced

6 slices bacon, cooked and crumbled

1 stalk celery, diced

8 oz. mushrooms, sliced

3 red onions, sliced

2 carrots, diced

Ghee

Ground black pepper

Sea salt

## *Instructions:*

a. Set an oven to 425 degrees.

b. Sprinkle black pepper and salt over the squash and bake it for about 45 minutes. Scrape the flesh from the squash once cooked and set aside.

c.  Using a skillet, sauté 1 onion, celery, garlic and carrots in ghee over medium-high heat for about 5 minutes.

d.  Add cinnamon and beef. Once meat is brown, add mushrooms.

e.  Remove the skillet from heat once vegetables are tender.

f.  Add squash to the beef mixture and mix well. Cook in the oven for about 10 minutes.

g.  Once done cooking, place equal amounts of the beef mixture in the squash shells.

h.  In a separate skillet, sauté remaining onions in ghee until caramelized.

i.  Place onions together with bacon on top of the squash as garnishes.

# *Dessert: Fruit Juice Gelatin*

Number of Servings: 4

## *Ingredients:*

4 cups of preferred fruit juice

1 cup fresh berries, assorted

4 tablespoons gelatin powder


## *Instructions:*

a.  Place 3 cups of fruit juice in a pan and bring it to boil.

b.  Dissolve gelatin powder in the remaining bowl of fruit juice. Stir well.

c.  Pour hot juice into the gelatin mixture and mix well.

d.  Transfer the mixture into a pan.

e.  Distribute mixed berries evenly into the mixture.

f.  Refrigerate the mixture for a minimum of 3 hours.

## *Snack: Almond and Apple Butter Bites*

### *Ingredients:*

1 apple

Dried cranberries

Almond butter

Dark chocolate chips

Pecans, chopped

Coconut shreds, roasted

Almonds, sliced

### *Instructions:*

a.   Remove the core of the apple and slice it thinly.

b.   Smear almond butter over one side of each slice of apple.

c.   Spread remaining ingredients on top of each slice.

# CHAPTER 7

# Day Six

## *Breakfast: Sweet Potato and Sausage Casserole*

Number of Servings: 8 to 10

### *Ingredients:*

1 ½ lbs. breakfast sausage

4 cups kale

¼ cup coconut milk

12 eggs, whisked

1 teaspoon pepper

2 sweet potatoes, peeled and diced

1 teaspoon sea salt

½ large sweet onion, diced

¼ teaspoon nutmeg

1 teaspoon garlic powder

Coconut oil

## *Instructions:*

a. Set the oven to 375 degrees. Use coconut oil to grease a 9x13 casserole dish.

b. Grease a skillet with coconut oil and place it over medium heat.

c. Add sausage into the skillet and break it down using a wooden spoon. Cook until brown.

d. Put onions and sweet potatoes together in a food processor and shred. Once done, transfer contents into a large bowl.

e. Add remaining ingredients into the bowl and mix well.

f. Pour the egg mixture into the casserole dish. Add cooked sausage and distribute evenly.

g. Place casserole in the oven and bake for about 45 minutes.

h. Once done, cover the casserole dish with foil and bake for another 10 minutes.

## *Lunch: Chicken and Avocado Salad*

Number of Servings: 4

### *Ingredients:*

4 skinless chicken thighs, deboned

½ red onion, diced

1 teaspoon chili powder

2 small tomatoes, diced

1 teaspoon cumin

1 teaspoon sea salt

3 avocado, peeled and seeded

1 tablespoon avocado oil

Lime juice

Black pepper


### *Instructions:*

a.  Set the oven to 350 degrees.

b.  Place chicken thighs side-by-side in a glass baking dish.

c.  Sprinkle cumin, chili powder, salt and oil on top.

d.  Bake chicken for about 30 minutes or until cooked through.

e.  Place avocado in a bowl and mash it lightly using a fork.

f.  Add onion, chicken and tomato. Drizzle with lime juice and stir well. Season to taste.

# Dinner: Pineapple and Pork Stir-Fry

Number of Servings: 4

## Ingredients:

1 ½ lbs. pork tenderloin

1 tablespoon tapioca starch

1 large bell pepper, chopped

2 cloves garlic, minced

1 onion, chopped

1-inch piece ginger, minced

20 oz. pineapple

¼ cup pineapple juice

¼ cup coconut aminos

Sea salt

Ghee

Ground black pepper

## Instructions:

a. Slice pork and pineapple into chunks.

b. Fry pork in ghee using a skillet for about 5 minutes. Stir continuously.

c. Remove from heat once done and set aside.

d.  Place ginger, garlic and onion in the skillet. Sauté for about 2 minutes.

e.  Add pineapple and bell pepper. Once slightly tender, pour pineapple juice and coconut aminos into the mixture.

f.  Place the pork back in the skillet. Add tapioca starch and stir well to combine.

## *Dessert: Fruit Cake*

Number of Servings: 8 to 10

### *Ingredients:*

1 ½ cups almond flour

½ teaspoon sea salt

½ cup tapioca flour

1 cup preferred dry fruits, assorted

½ teaspoon baking powder

1 cup dried cherries

5 eggs

2 cups raisins

1 cup honey, raw

1 cup dates, chopped

1 cup ghee

1 teaspoon vanilla extract

1 teaspoon cloves, ground

1 teaspoon nutmeg, ground

1 teaspoon cinnamon, ground

## Instructions:

a. Heat an oven to 350 degrees beforehand. Grease a loaf pan using non-stick cooking spray.

b. Put almond flour, salt, tapioca flour and baking powder in a bowl. Mix well.

c. Add cloves, nutmeg and cinnamon into the mixture. Combine ingredients thoroughly.

d. Whisk eggs, honey, butter and vanilla together in a separate bowl.

e. Combine the two mixtures together. Mix until smooth.

f. Add dried fruits and stir well until evenly distributed.

g. Pour the mixture into the loaf pan and place it in the oven. Cook for about an hour.

# Snack: Raspberry, Watermelon and Mint Salad

## Ingredients:

½ cup hazelnuts

¼ cup lime juice

¼ cup mint, shredded

1 cup raspberries

1/3 cup water

1 tablespoon honey, raw

1 ½ cups strawberries, hulled and sliced

½ small watermelon

## Instructions:

a. Set an oven to 350 degrees.

b. Place the hazelnuts on a baking tray and place it in the oven. Cook for about 10 minutes.

c. Once done, remove the skins from the nuts. Chop coarsely.

d. Combine water, honey and lime juice together in a saucepan. Warm the mixture up over low heat for about 5 minutes then set aside.

e. Remove the rind of the watermelon and discard. Cut flesh into chunks and place these in a bowl together with raspberries, mint and strawberries.

f. Pour liquid mixture over the fruits and mix gently. Garnish with nuts.

# CHAPTER 8

# Day Seven

## *Breakfast: Egg in a Jar*

Number of Servings: 4

### *Ingredients:*

4 large eggs

1 tablespoon ghee

¾ lb. button mushrooms, sliced thinly

2 teaspoons lemon juice

4 slices bacon

½ cup chicken stock

2 green onions, minced

1 teaspoon almond flour

1 tablespoon chives, minced

Ground black pepper

Sea salt

## Instructions:

a. Cut bacon into chunks.

b. Using a skillet, cook bacon in ghee over medium-high heat for about 10 minutes.

c. Add green onions and mushrooms into the skillet and cook for another 5 minutes.

d. Add almond flour and mix well. Pour chicken stock together with lemon juice into the mixture.

e. Bring mixture into a boil and cook until smooth.

f. Grease the insides of 4 glass jars using ghee. Transfer equal amounts of the bacon mixture into each jar.

g. Crack an egg on top of each. Season with black pepper and salt.

h. Put the jars into a cooking pot. Pour water into the pot until it covers half of the jars.

i. Place the pot over medium-high heat and cook for about 20 minutes.

j. Remove the jars from the pot once done. Garnish with chives.

# Lunch: Thai Pork Lettuce Wraps

Number of Servings: 4

## Ingredients:

1 lb. pork, sliced thinly

1 tablespoon ghee

2 cups chicken stock

1 lime, quartered

2 tablespoons white wine vinegar

¾ lb. mung bean sprouts

1 teaspoon sambal sauce

½ cup almond butter

4 tablespoons water

1 tablespoon fish sauce

Fresh lettuce leaves

Ground black pepper

Sea salt

## Instructions:

a. Pour chicken stock into a pan. Bring it to a boil over medium-high heat.

b. Add pork and cook gently for about 5 minutes.

c. Once cooked, transfer the pork into a plate and set aside to cool. Pour chicken stock into a separate bowl and refrigerate for later recipes.

d. Grease a pan using ghee. Add bean sprouts and cook for about 4 minutes.

e. Combine all of the remaining ingredients together in a bowl except for lettuce leaves and mix well.

f. Cut lettuce leaves into 3x3-inch pieces. Distribute pork, bean sprouts and almond butter mixture into each leaf.

g. Drizzle with lime juice on top of each and roll into wraps.

# *Dinner: Stuffed Calamari*

Number of Servings: 4

## *Ingredients:*

4 large calamari

14 oz. tomato puree

5 oz. kale, chopped

1 onion, minced

1 teaspoon dried oregano

1 red bell pepper, chopped

2 tablespoons parsley, chopped finely

2 cloves garlic, minced

Ghee

Ground black pepper

Sea salt

## *Instructions:*

a. Remove the tentacles from the calamari. Chop these finely and set aside.

b. Using a skillet, sauté onions and garlic in ghee over medium heat. Add bell peppers and continue cooking.

c. After 3 minutes, put tentacles in the skillet and cook for another 8 minutes.

d.  Add kale and cook until soft. Stir frequently while cooking and remove from heat once done.

e.  Divide the mixture into 4 equal amounts and use it to stuff each calamari. Use toothpicks to close up each calamari.

f.  Put some ghee in the skillet and place it over medium-high heat.

g.  Cook each side of the calamari for about 2 minutes. Add tomato puree together with oregano and parsley. Stir gently and season to taste.

h.  Reduce the heat and bring mixture to a simmer. Cover the pan and cook for about 40 minutes.

i.  Adjust seasoning if necessary.

# *Dessert: Fruit Pudding*

Number of Servings: 4

## *Ingredients:*

1 lb. frozen fruit of choice

5 tablespoons tapioca starch

2 cups orange juice

4 mint leaves

## *Instructions:*

a. Put orange juice and fruits in a saucepan and place it over medium heat. Bring it to a simmer.

b. After a few minutes, use a fine mesh sieve to strain the mixture.

c. Transfer the fruit residue in a separate bowl and place it in the refrigerator.

d. Bring the fruit juice to a simmer. Using a ladle, pour a portion of the fruit juice in a bowl.

e. Add water and tapioca starch into the bowl and mix well.

f. Once combined thoroughly, pour the fruit juice mixture back into the saucepan and stir well until thick.

g. Distribute the mixture evenly into 4 glasses. Refrigerate for at least 2 hours or overnight.

h. Garnish with extra fruit slices and mint leaves.

## *Snack: Fruit Salad with Lime*

### *Ingredients:*

1 cup red grapes, seedless

8 strips lime peel

1 cup green grapes, seedless

1 teaspoon lime zest

3 plums

2 tablespoons mint, minced

2 peaches, peeled

2 tablespoons lime juice

2 nectarines

6 sprigs mint

1 cup water

### *Instructions:*

a.  Slice plum, nectarines and peaches into wedges.

b.  Pour water into a small saucepan together with mint sprigs and lime peel. Cook the mixture and reduce it to half.

c.  Discard the mint sprigs and lime peel. Set aside the mixture to cool.

d.  Add mint, lime juice and lime zest.

e. Place red grapes, nectarines, green grapes, peaches and plums in a bowl. Mix well.

f. Drizzle sauce over the fruits and mix gently.

# CHAPTER 9

# Condiments

## *Ketchup Recipes*

Simple Ketchup

*Ingredients:*

6 oz. tomato paste

1/8 teaspoon cayenne pepper

2 tablespoons lemon juice or vinegar

1 pinch allspice, ground

¼ teaspoon dry mustard

1 pinch cloves, ground

1/3 cup water

¼ teaspoon salt

¼ teaspoon cinnamon


*Instructions:*

a.   Place all of the ingredients in a bowl. Mix well.

# *Deep-flavored Ketchup*

## *Ingredients:*

2 lbs. plum tomatoes, chopped

¾ cup balsamic vinegar

1 large onion, chopped

1 teaspoon ground black pepper

½ bulb fennel, chopped

2 cloves garlic, chopped

1 stick celery, diced

1 tablespoon coriander seeds

1-inch piece ginger

½ red chili, seeded and chopped

1 ½ cups water

Bunch of basil

Extra virgin olive oil

Sea salt

## *Instructions:*

a.  Separate the basil leaves from the stalks. Chop the stalks finely.

b.  Combine onion, garlic, fennel, coriander, celery, basil stalks, olive oil, chili and ginger together in a sauce pan. Season to taste.

c. Cook for about 12 minutes over low heat. Stir occasionally.

d. Add tomatoes and water into the mixture. Cook gently until reduced by half.

e. Add basil leaves and transfer the mixture into a food processor. Blend until smooth.

f. Filter the sauce using a sieve and add vinegar.

g. Place the mixture in a saucepan. Cooked gently until preferred texture is obtained.

h. Adjust seasoning as necessary.

# *Chunky Apple Ketchup*

## *Ingredients:*

24 red tomatoes, diced and peeled

2 tablespoon pickling spices

8 apples, seeded, peeled and diced

1 cup honey, raw

2 bell peppers, diced, and seeded

2 pears, seeded, peeled and diced

1 cup apple cider vinegar

4 onions, diced

Sea salt

## *Instructions:*

a. Wrap the pickling spices using a piece of cheesecloth. Tie tightly to close.

b. Including the wrapped spices, place all of the ingredients in a large saucepan.

c. Bring the mixture to a boil over medium-high heat. Stir frequently.

d. Reduce heat to medium. Allow mixture to cook gently and uncovered for about an hour. Stir occasionally.

e. Discard the wrapped spices and transfer the ketchup into hot jars.

f.    Allow to cool. Store in the refrigerator once ready.

# *Mustard Recipes*

<u>Simple Mustard</u>

## *Ingredients:*

½ cup mustard powder

Sea salt

½ cup water

2 tablespoons vinegar

Basil, chopped

Lemon zest


## *Instructions:*

a. Dissolve mustard powder in water.

b. Add remaining ingredients and mix well until combined thoroughly.

c. Let it sit for about 15 minutes.

# *Whole-Grain Mustard*

## *Ingredients:*

¼ cup yellow mustard seeds

½ teaspoon sea salt

4 teaspoons mustard powder

¼ cup brown mustard seeds

¼ cup white wine vinegar

1 cup water

## *Instructions:*

a.  Place mustard seeds in a bowl together with water. Allow to soak overnight.

b.  Pour the contents of the bowl into a food processor together with remaining ingredients. Blend until thick.

c.  Transfer into a glass jar and put a lid on it. Place it in the refrigerator for 4 days.

Additional Tip: you can also experiment with this recipe by adding sun-dried tomatoes, fresh herbs and/or fresh basil.

# *Horseradish Recipes*

<u>Simple Horseradish</u>

## *Ingredients:*

1 cup horseradish root, peeled and minced

¼ teaspoon sea salt

¾ cup white wine vinegar

## *Instructions:*

a.  Place all of the ingredients in a food processor and blend until thick.

# *Beet Horseradish*

## *Ingredients:*

¾ lb. horseradish root, minced

¾ cup apple cider vinegar

1 cup beets, chopped finely

½ teaspoon sea salt

## *Instructions:*

a.  Lace all of the ingredients in a food processor and blend until thick.

## *Traditional Fermented Horseradish*

### *Ingredients:*

1 cup horseradish root, peeled and chopped finely

4 tablespoons water

1 packet vegetable culture starter

1 ½ teaspoon sea salt

### *Instructions:*

a.  Place horseradish root, sea salt and starter culture in a food processor. Blend until combined thoroughly.

b.  Add water and blend for about 3 minutes.

c.  Transfer horseradish paste into a small glass jar. Fill the jar with extra water.

d.  Place the lid loosely and set aside for 3 to 7 days in a warm place. Refrigerate once done.

# *Worcestershire Sauce*

## *Ingredients:*

½ cup apple cider vinegar

1/8 teaspoon ground black pepper

2 tablespoons water

1/8 teaspoon cinnamon

2 tablespoon coconut aminos

¼ teaspoon garlic powder

¼ teaspoon ginger, ground

¼ teaspoon onion powder

¼ teaspoon mustard powder

## *Instructions:*

a.  Place all of the ingredients in a saucepan and mix well.

b.  Allow to cook while stirring frequently and bring it to a boil.

c.  Cook gently for another minute. Set aside to cool. Refrigerate.

# *Barbecue Sauce*

## *Ingredients:*

1 onion, minced

1 pinch cinnamon

1 clove garlic, minced

1 pinch cloves, ground

6 oz. tomato paste

¼ cup homemade ketchup

1 tablespoon Worcestershire sauce

½ cup apple cider vinegar

3 tablespoons homemade mustard

½ cup water

Paprika, smoked

## *Instructions:*

a. Using a large skillet, sauté onion in ghee for about 4 minutes.

b. Add garlic and continue sautéing for 1 more minute.

c. Add remaining ingredients and cook gently for half an hour.

d. Season with paprika and adjust seasoning as necessary.

e. Set aside to cool. Refrigerate.

# *Mayonnaise Recipes*

<u>Simple Mayonnaise</u>

## *Ingredients:*

2 egg yolks

1 pinch salt

1 cup light olive oil

4 teaspoon lemon juice

1 tablespoon homemade or Dijon mustard

## *Instructions:*

a. Put egg yolks, mustard, 1 teaspoon of lemon juice and salt in a food processor.

b. Blend the ingredients together while gradually and steadily adding the oil.

c. Once mixture is thick, add remaining lemon juice and blend well.

# *Coconut Mayonnaise*

## *Ingredients:*

2 eggs yolks

½ cup coconut oil

1 teaspoon mustard

½ cup olive oil

3 teaspoon lemon juice

## *Instructions:*

a.  Put yolks, 1 teaspoon of lemon juice and mustard in a food processor.

b.  Blend the mixture continuously while gradually adding the oil.

c.  Once mixture is thick, add remaining lemon juice and stir well. Season with ground black pepper and salt if desired.

Additional Tip: You can use 1 cup of liquid bacon fat instead of coconut and olive oils to create a baconnaise version of this recipe.

# *Salsa Recipes*

## Fire-Roasted Salsa

### *Ingredients:*

2 lbs. Roma tomatoes

½ teaspoon oregano

1 jalapeno pepper

¼ teaspoon cumin

½ bunch cilantro

1 large white onion, sliced

1 tablespoon lime juice

3 cloves garlic, minced

Ground black pepper

Sea salt

### *Instructions:*

a. Set a grill to medium-high heat beforehand.

b. On a baking sheet, arrange tomatoes, jalapeno, onion and garlic in a single layer.

c. Cook the vegetables in the grill for about 10 to 15 minutes on each side.

d. Place the grilled vegetables in a food processor and blend until desired texture is obtained.

e. Pour salsa into a bowl together with remaining ingredients. Stir well.

# *Melon Salsa*

## *Ingredients:*

1 cup watermelon, chopped

2 tablespoons cilantro, minced

1 cup cantaloupe, chopped

½ avocado, chopped

1 cup honeydew melon, chopped

¼ red onion, chopped

½ cucumber, chopped and seeded

Lime juice

Ground black pepper

Sea salt

## *Instructions:*

a.  Place watermelon, cucumber, avocado, cantaloupe, onion and honeydew together in a bowl. Mix well.

b.  Add remaining ingredients and stir well.

# *Mexican Salsa Verde*

## *Ingredients:*

½ cup onion, chopped

2 jalapeno peppers, chopped and seeded

1 ½ lb. green tomatillos

2 tablespoons lime juice

½ cup cilantro, chopped

Salt

Ground black pepper

## *Instructions:*

a.  Remove the husks of the tomatillos and slice each fruit lengthwise.

b.  Roast the tomatillos on a grill for about 6 minutes.

c.  Place all of the ingredients in a blender. Process until smooth.

# *Sweet Potato Hummus*

## *Ingredients:*

4 cups sweet potatoes, peeled

¼ teaspoon cayenne pepper

2 cloves garlic, minced

¼ cup tahini

2 teaspoons cumin, ground

¼ cup lime juice

Ground black pepper

Sea salt

## *Instructions:*

a.   Slice the sweet potatoes into big chunks.

b.   Pour water with salted into a pot and add sweet potatoes. Cook gently for about 10 minutes.

c.   Remove excess water. Transfer the sweet potato into a bowl and use a fork to mash it. Refrigerate.

d.   Once cooled, add all of the remaining ingredients into the sweet potato mash.

e.   Stir well and adjust seasoning as needed.

Additional Tip: Tahini is a simple nut butter that is made from sesame seeds. To make one, you just have to roast 1 cup of sesame seeds at 350 degrees in a preheated oven for about 8 minutes. Make sure to shake the seeds frequently while cooking. Afterwards, transfer the sesame seeds to a food processor together with olive oil and blend for about 5 minutes.

# *Sriracha Sauce*

## *Ingredients:*

1 ½ lbs. Fresno or jalapeno peppers, seeded and stemmed

2 tablespoons extra virgin olive oil

4 Thai chilies, seeded and stemmed

2 tablespoons fish sauce

2 tablespoons tomato paste

5 cloves garlic

2 tablespoons honey, raw

3 tablespoons white wine vinegar

Sea salt

## *Ingredients:*

a. Chop the jalapeno roughly and slice the Thai chilies thinly. Place them in a blender together with garlic.

b. Place all of the ingredients in the blender and process until smooth. Season to taste then transfer the sauce into a pan.

c. Place the pan over medium-high heat and bring the sauce into a boil. Decrease the heat to low.

d. Cook gently for about 10 minutes. Stir occasionally.

e. Store the sauce in a jar once cooled.

# *Basil Pesto*

## *Ingredients:*

2 cups basil leaves

3 cloves garlic, minced

½ cup extra virgin olive oil

1/3 cup pine nuts

Ground black pepper

Sea salt

## *Instructions:*

a.  Combine garlic, basil and nuts together in a food processor. Pulse until ingredients are chopped.

b.  Add olive oil and process again until smooth. Season to taste.

Additional Tip: If pine nuts are not immediately available, you can use walnuts or cashews as replacement.

# Conclusion

Paleo diet is extremely easy to follow. Its dishes are also extremely delicious making it easy to stick to your food regimen. Not only will it help you attain your fitness goals but your new eating habits will also aid you to become healthier and avoid medical conditions such as hypertension and obesity.

Thank you again for purchasing this book!

I hope this book was able to help you to create delicious dishes that can help you start your paleo diet.

The next step is to continue eating paleo-approved dishes and food products to maintain your health goals.

Finally, if you enjoyed this book, then I'd like to ask you for a favor, would you be kind enough to leave a review for this book on Amazon? It'd be greatly appreciated!

Thank you and good luck!

www.ingramcontent.com/pod-product-compliance
Lightning Source LLC
Chambersburg PA
CBHW060152290526
45789CB00003B/1010